Parkinson's Disease Diet Cookbook For Beginners

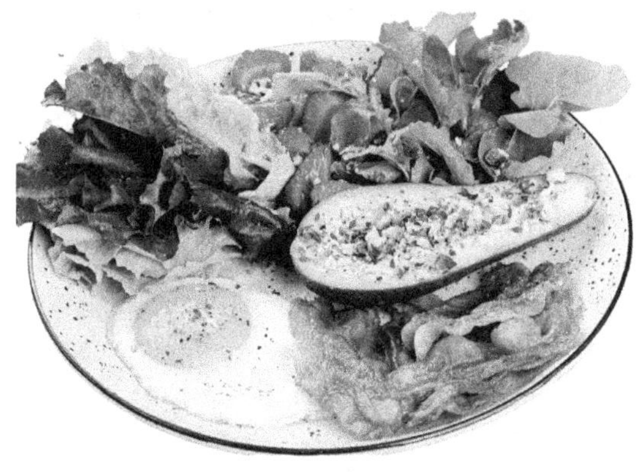

A Guide to Healthy and Delicious Recipes for Every Stage of the Disease to Boost Your Brain and Body.

Dr.Rebecca J. Reynolds

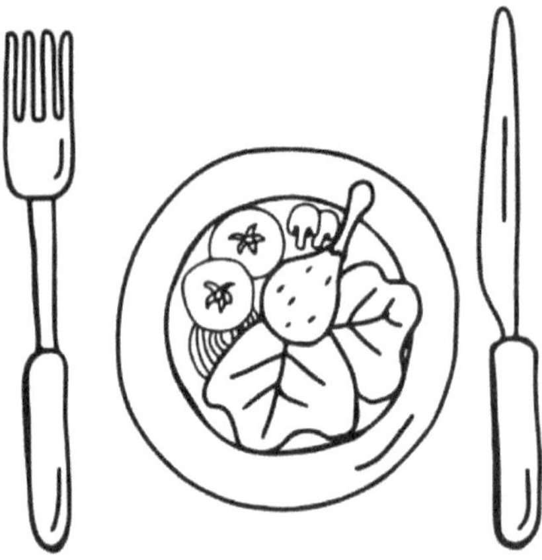

Table Of Content

DINNER

Spaghetti with whole-wheat pasta, turkey meatballs, and marinara sauce

Vegetable stir-fry with brown rice, tofu, and soy sauce

Salmon with lemon, garlic, and rosemary, served with mashed potatoes and broccoli

Chicken and vegetable casserole with cream of mushroom soup and cheese

Lentil and vegetable curry with coconut milk and naan bread

SNACKS

Trail mix with nuts, dried fruits, and dark chocolate

Yogurt with granola and fresh berries

Carrot sticks with hummus and whole-wheat crackers

Popcorn with olive oil and sea salt

Apple slices with peanut butter and raisins

Part 2:

Recipes for Moderate Stage Parkinson's & Advanced Stage Parkinson's

Breakfast

Banana waffles

Berry smoothie

Apple muffins

Cereal with almond milk, nuts, and dried fruits

Egg and cheese quiche with whole-wheat crust, spinach, and mushrooms

LUNCH

Chicken burger

INTRODUCTION

Parkinson's disease is a progressive neurological disorder that affects the movement, balance, and coordination of millions of people worldwide. It is caused by the loss of dopamine-producing cells in the brain, which leads to symptoms such as tremors, stiffness, slowness, and difficulty with walking, speaking, and swallowing. Parkinson's disease can also affect the mood, memory, sleep, and digestion of people living with the condition.

While there is no cure for Parkinson's disease, there are treatments and therapies that can help manage the symptoms and improve the quality of life of people with Parkinson's disease. One of the most important aspects of living well with Parkinson's disease is diet and nutrition. What you eat and drink can have a significant impact on your brain and body, and can either help or worsen your symptoms.

In this book, you will learn how to eat well with Parkinson's disease, and how to prepare healthy and delicious recipes for every stage of the disease. You will discover the benefits of eating foods that are rich in antioxidants, omega-3s, fiber, magnesium, and probiotics, and how to avoid foods that are high in fat, sugar, or processed ingredients. You will also learn how to time your meals and snacks according to your medication schedule, and how to overcome common challenges such as swallowing difficulty, constipation, weight loss, or loss of appetite.

This book contains over 100 recipes for breakfast, lunch, dinner, snacks, and desserts, that are easy to make, nutritious, and tasty. Each recipe includes the nutritional information, serving size, cooking time, and step-by-step instructions. You will find recipes for oatmeal, smoothies, eggs, pancakes, muffins, salads, sandwiches, soups, wraps, bowls, pasta, rice, curry, stir-fry, casserole, granola bars, cookies, cakes, pies, and more. All the recipes are designed to boost your brain and body, and to suit your preferences and tastes.

Whether you are newly diagnosed with Parkinson's disease, or you have been living with it for years, this book will help you enjoy food and nourish your health. By following the guidelines and recipes in this book, you will be able to eat well, feel well, and live well with Parkinson's disease.

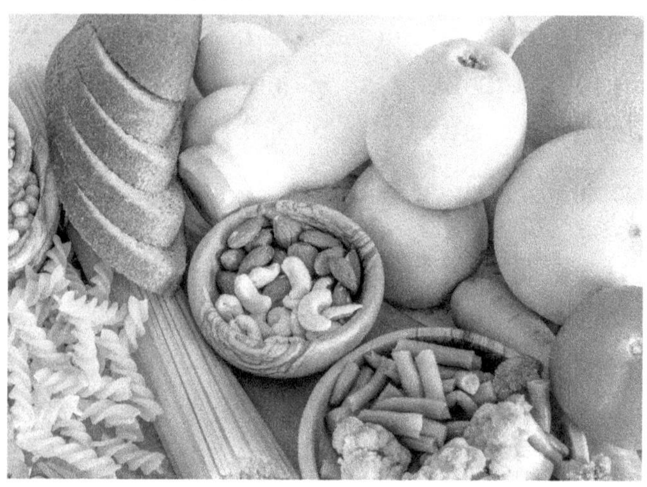

What is Parkinson's disease and how does it affect your body and brain

Parkinson's disease is a brain disorder that causes problems with movement, balance, and other functions. It happens when certain nerve cells in the brain die or become damaged. These cells produce a chemical called dopamine, which helps control muscle activity and coordination. Without enough dopamine, the brain cannot send the right signals to the muscles, leading to tremors, stiffness, slowness, and other symptoms. Parkinson's disease can also affect other parts of the brain that are involved in mood, memory, thinking, and digestion. There is no cure for Parkinson's disease, but treatments can help manage the symptoms and improve the quality of life for people with the condition.

Why is diet important for managing Parkinson's symptoms and complications

Diet is important for managing Parkinson's symptoms and complications because it can affect your body and brain in various ways. Some of the benefits of a healthy diet for people with Parkinson's are:

It can help you maintain a normal body weight, which can reduce the risk of other health problems, such as diabetes, heart disease, and osteoporosis.

It can provide you with enough energy, protein, vitamins, minerals, and fiber to support your immune system, muscle function, bone health, and digestion.

It can help you avoid or reduce constipation, which is a common and bothersome symptom of Parkinson's that can affect your quality of life and medication absorption.

It can help you optimize the effects of your medications, by avoiding foods that may interfere with their absorption or cause side effects, such as nausea or low blood pressure.

It can help you prevent or delay cognitive decline, by including foods that are rich in antioxidants, omega-3 fatty acids, and other nutrients that protect your brain cells and enhance your memory and thinking .

Therefore, following a balanced and varied diet that includes plenty of whole foods, such as fruits, vegetables, whole grains, lean protein, nuts, seeds, and healthy fats, can improve your overall health and well-being with Parkinson's.

What are the general principles of a healthy Parkinson's diet

A healthy Parkinson's diet is one that can help you manage your symptoms, prevent complications, and improve your overall well-being. Some of the general principles of a healthy Parkinson's diet are:

Eat a balanced diet with a variety of foods from all the food groups, such as vegetables, fruits, whole grains, lean protein, nuts, seeds, and healthy fats.

Drink plenty of water and fluids to stay hydrated and avoid constipation, which is a common problem for people with Parkinson's .

Get enough fiber from foods like fruits, vegetables, beans, and whole grains to improve your digestion and bowel movements.

Avoid or limit foods that may interfere with your medication absorption or cause side effects, such as iron, protein, citrus juices, alcohol, and caffeine .

Include foods that are rich in antioxidants, omega-3 fatty acids, and other nutrients that can protect your brain cells and slow down cognitive decline, such as berries, fish, nuts, and olive oil.

Tips for Dealing with Swallowing Difficulties

Swallowing difficulties and digestion issues are common problems for people with Parkinson's disease. They can affect your nutrition, hydration, and quality of life. Here are some tips for dealing with these challenges:

- See a speech and language therapist. They can assess your swallowing function and recommend exercises, strategies, and modifications to help you eat and drink safely and comfortably.
- Choose soft, moist, and easy-to-chew foods. Avoid hard, dry, or crumbly foods that can be difficult to swallow or cause choking. You can also puree your food in a blender or use a liquid thickener to make thin liquids easier to swallow.
- Eat small, frequent meals. This can help you get enough calories and nutrients without feeling too full or bloated. It can also reduce the risk of acid reflux, which can worsen your swallowing and digestion problems.

- Drink plenty of fluids. This can help you stay hydrated, prevent constipation, and lubricate your throat. Aim for at least eight glasses of water a day, and avoid caffeinated, carbonated, or alcoholic drinks that can dehydrate you or irritate your stomach.
- Chew well and swallow carefully. Cut your food into small pieces, and chew it thoroughly before swallowing. Don't talk with food in your mouth, and eat slowly. Swallow one mouthful before taking the next, and use a spoon or fork rather than a straw.
- Sit upright and stay focused. Have your meal in a quiet place, and reduce distractions. Sit upright during meal times, and remain upright for at least 30 minutes after. Do not lie down or recline after eating, as this can increase the risk of aspiration or reflux.
- Take your medication as prescribed. Some medications can help improve your swallowing and digestion, such as levodopa, domperidone, or laxatives.

Follow your doctor's instructions on when and how to take them, and let them know if you have any side effects or concerns

How to use this cookbook: tips, tools, and resources

This cookbook is designed to help you prepare healthy and delicious recipes for every stage of Parkinson's disease. Here are some tips, tools, and resources to help you use this cookbook effectively:

- Read the introduction section to learn more about Parkinson's disease, its symptoms, complications, and the importance of diet for managing the condition.

- Browse the three parts of the cookbook, each corresponding to a different stage of Parkinson's: early, moderate, and advanced. Choose the recipes that suit your needs and preferences, and adjust them as necessary.
- Follow the instructions and measurements carefully for each recipe, and use the photos as a guide. You can also use a kitchen scale, measuring cups, spoons, and a thermometer to ensure accuracy and safety.
- Use the ingredient list to check what you have in your pantry, fridge, or freezer, and what you need to buy. You can also use the nutrition facts to track your calories, carbs, protein, fat, and other nutrients.

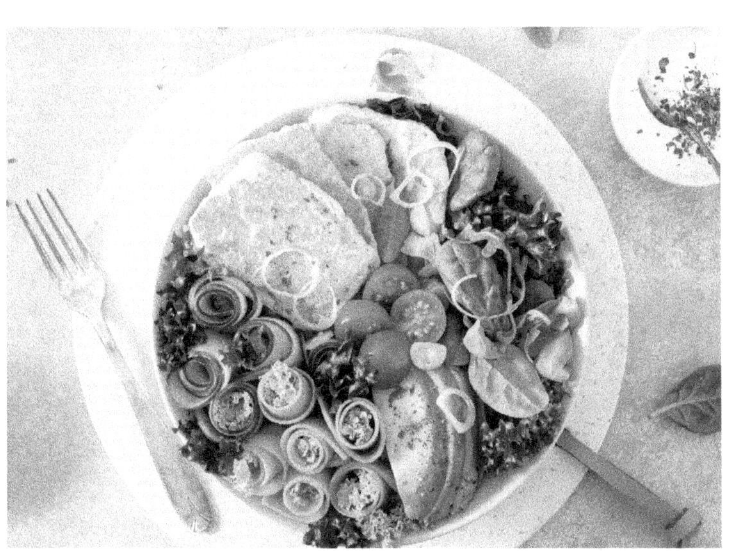

Part 1:

Recipes for Early Stage Parkinson's

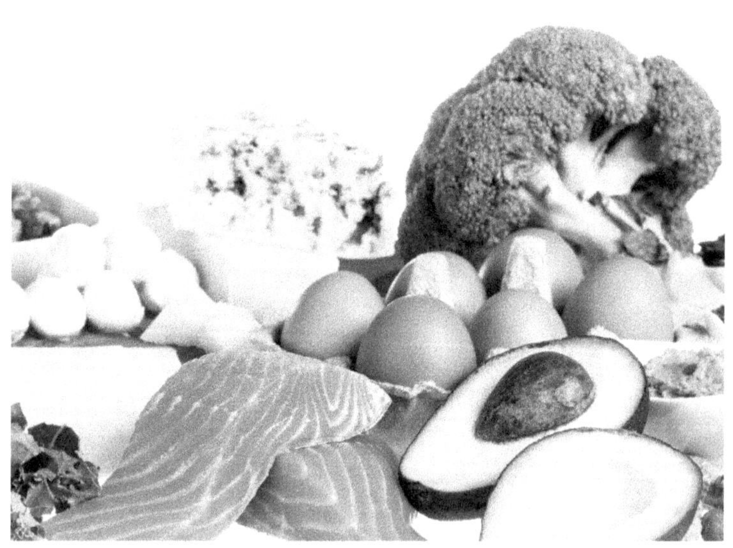

Breakfast

Oatmeal with Blueberries, Walnuts, and Honey

Ingredients

- 1 cup of rolled oats
- 2 cups of water
- A pinch of salt
- 1/4 cup of fresh or frozen blueberries
- 2 tablespoons of chopped walnuts
- 2 tablespoons of honey

Instructions

1. In a small saucepan, bring the water and salt to a boil over high heat.
2. Add the oats and reduce the heat to medium-low. Simmer, stirring occasionally, for about 15 minutes or until the oats are soft and creamy.
3. Stir in the blueberries and cook for another 5 minutes or until they are warm and burst.

4. Divide the oatmeal into two bowls and top with the walnuts and honey. Enjoy!

Serving Size

- This recipe makes 2 servings.
- Each serving is about 1 cup of oatmeal.

Nutritional Content

- Per serving: 345 calories, 11 g fat, 2 g saturated fat, 0 mg cholesterol, 75 mg sodium, 58 g carbohydrates, 7 g fiber, 25 g sugar, 9 g protein.

Banana Smoothie with Almond Milk, Yogurt, and Flax Seeds

Ingredients

- 1 large ripe banana, peeled and sliced
- 1 cup of unsweetened almond milk
- 1/2 cup of plain Greek yogurt
- 2 tablespoons of ground flax seeds

- 1 teaspoon of vanilla extract
- A few ice cubes

Instructions

1. In a blender, combine the banana, almond milk, yogurt, flax seeds, and vanilla. Blend until smooth and creamy.
2. Add the ice cubes and blend again until frosty.
3. Pour the smoothie into a large glass and enjoy!

Serving Size

- This recipe makes 1 serving.
- Each serving is about 2 cups of smoothie.

Nutritional Content

- Per serving: 365 calories, 14 g fat, 2 g saturated fat, 5 mg cholesterol, 180 mg sodium, 51 g carbohydrates, 10 g fiber, 29 g sugar, 16 g protein.

Scrambled Eggs with Spinach, Cheese, and Whole-Wheat Toast

Ingredients

- 4 large eggs
- 1/4 cup of milk
- Salt and pepper to taste
- 1 tablespoon of butter
- 2 cups of baby spinach
- 1/4 cup of shredded cheddar cheese
- 4 slices of whole-wheat bread
- Optional: jam, butter, or honey for the toast

Instructions

1. In a medium bowl, whisk the eggs, milk, salt, and pepper until well combined.
2. In a large skillet over medium-high heat, melt the butter and swirl to coat the pan.
3. Add the spinach and cook, stirring occasionally, for about 5 minutes or until wilted.

4. Reduce the heat to low and pour the egg mixture over the spinach. Cook, stirring gently, for about 10 minutes or until the eggs are set and fluffy.
5. Sprinkle the cheese over the eggs and cover the pan with a lid. Cook for another 5 minutes or until the cheese is melted.
6. Meanwhile, toast the bread in a toaster or oven until golden and crisp.
7. Serve the scrambled eggs with the toast and your choice of jam, butter, or honey. Enjoy!

Serving Size

- This recipe makes 4 servings.
- Each serving is 1/4 of the scrambled eggs and 1 slice of toast.

Nutritional Content

- Per serving: 295 calories, 17 g fat, 8 g saturated fat, 223 mg cholesterol, 343 mg sodium, 21 g carbohydrates, 3 g fiber, 5 g sugar, 16 g protein.

Apple Cinnamon Pancakes with Maple Syrup and Almond Butter

Ingredients

- 1 1/2 cups of whole-wheat flour
- 2 teaspoons of baking powder
- 1/4 teaspoon of salt
- 1 teaspoon of cinnamon
- 1 1/4 cups of milk
- 2 eggs
- 2 tablespoons of melted butter
- 1/4 cup of maple syrup
- 1 apple, peeled, cored, and grated
- 1/4 cup of almond butter

Instructions

1. In a large bowl, whisk together the flour, baking powder, salt, and cinnamon.
2. In a medium bowl, whisk together the milk, eggs, butter, and 2 tablespoons of maple syrup.

3. Add the wet ingredients to the dry ingredients and stir until just combined. Fold in the grated apple.
4. Heat a lightly greased griddle or skillet over medium-high heat. Drop 1/4 cup of batter onto the griddle and cook for about 3 minutes or until bubbles form on the surface. Flip and cook for another 2 minutes or until golden and cooked through. Repeat with the remaining batter.
5. Serve the pancakes with the remaining maple syrup and almond butter. Enjoy!

Serving Size

- This recipe makes 12 pancakes.
- Each serving is 2 pancakes.

Nutritional Content

- Per serving: 315 calories, 13 g fat, 4 g saturated fat, 68 mg cholesterol, 234 mg sodium, 43 g carbohydrates, 6 g fiber, 18 g sugar, 10 g protein.

Berry Muffins with Oat Bran, Eggs, and Milk

Ingredients

- 1 1/2 cups of oat bran
- 1 cup of whole-wheat flour
- 1/4 cup of brown sugar
- 2 teaspoons of baking powder
- 1/2 teaspoon of salt
- 1 cup of milk
- 2 eggs
- 1/4 cup of vegetable oil
- 1 teaspoon of vanilla extract
- 1 cup of fresh or frozen mixed berries

Instructions

1. Preheat the oven to 375°F and line a 12-cup muffin tin with paper liners.
2. In a large bowl, whisk together the oat bran, flour, sugar, baking powder, and salt.
3. In a medium bowl, whisk together the milk, eggs, oil, and vanilla.

4. Add the wet ingredients to the dry ingredients and stir until just combined. Gently fold in the berries.
5. Spoon the batter into the prepared muffin cups, filling them about 3/4 full.
6. Bake for 18 to 20 minutes or until a toothpick inserted in the center comes out clean.
7. Let the muffins cool slightly in the pan before transferring them to a wire rack to cool completely.
8. Serve the muffins with butter, jam, or honey if desired. Enjoy!

Serving Size

- This recipe makes 12 muffins.
- Each serving is 1 muffin.

Nutritional Content

- Per serving: 185 calories, 8 g fat, 1 g saturated fat, 32 mg cholesterol, 174 mg sodium, 26 g carbohydrates, 4 g fiber, 9 g sugar, 6 g protein.

This is the end of the recipes for the breakfast dishes you listed. I hope you found them helpful and easy to follow. If you have any questions, feedback, or suggestions, please let me know. I'm always happy to help you.

LUNCH

Chicken Salad with Lettuce, Tomatoes, Cucumbers, and Avocado Dressing

Ingredients

- 2 cups of cooked chicken, shredded or chopped
- 4 cups of lettuce, torn or chopped
- 2 medium tomatoes, diced
- 1 large cucumber, peeled and sliced
- 1/4 cup of fresh parsley, chopped
- For the dressing:
    - 1 ripe avocado, peeled and pitted

  - 1/4 cup of plain yogurt
  - 2 tablespoons of lemon juice
  - 1 clove of garlic, minced
  - Salt and pepper to taste

Instructions

1. In a large bowl, toss the chicken, lettuce, tomatoes, cucumber, and parsley together. Set aside.
2. In a blender or food processor, combine the avocado, yogurt, lemon juice, garlic, salt, and pepper. Blend until smooth and creamy.
3. Drizzle the dressing over the salad and toss to coat. Serve immediately or refrigerate until ready to eat.

Serving Size

- This recipe makes 4 servings.
- Each serving is about 2 cups of salad.

Nutritional Content

- Per serving: 245 calories, 12 g fat, 3 g saturated fat, 63 mg cholesterol, 129 mg sodium, 13 g carbohydrates, 6 g fiber, 6 g sugar, 23 g protein.

Tomato Soup with Whole-Grain Bread and Cheese

Ingredients

- 2 tablespoons of olive oil
- 1 onion, chopped
- 2 cloves of garlic, minced
- 4 cups of vegetable broth
- 2 cans of diced tomatoes, with their juice
- 2 teaspoons of dried basil
- Salt and pepper to taste
- 4 slices of whole-grain bread
- 4 slices of cheddar cheese

Instructions

1. In a large pot over medium-high heat, heat the oil and cook the onion and garlic, stirring occasionally, for about 15 minutes or until soft and golden.

2. Add the broth, tomatoes, basil, salt, and pepper and bring to a boil. Reduce the heat and simmer, uncovered, for about 20 minutes or until slightly thickened.

3. Using an immersion blender or a food processor, puree the soup until smooth and creamy. You can also leave some chunks if you prefer a chunkier texture.

4. Preheat the oven to 375°F and line a baking sheet with parchment paper. Place the bread slices on the prepared sheet and top each with a cheese slice. Bake for 10 minutes or until the cheese is melted and bubbly.

5. Serve the soup with the cheese toast and enjoy!

Serving Size

- This recipe makes 4 servings.
- Each serving is about 1 1/2 cups of soup and 1 slice of cheese toast.

Nutritional Content

- Per serving: 365 calories, 19 g fat, 8 g saturated fat, 30 mg cholesterol, 857 mg

sodium, 37 g carbohydrates, 7 g fiber, 14 g
sugar, 14 g protein.

Turkey Wrap with Whole-Wheat Tortilla, Hummus, and Veggies

Ingredients

- 4 whole-wheat tortillas
- 1/2 cup of hummus
- 8 slices of turkey breast
- 2 cups of baby spinach
- 1/4 cup of shredded carrots
- 1/4 cup of sliced red onion
- Salt and pepper to taste

Instructions

1. Lay the tortillas on a flat surface and spread 2 tablespoons of hummus over each one.
2. Top each tortilla with 2 slices of turkey, 1/2 cup of spinach, 1 tablespoon of carrots, and 1 tablespoon of onion.
3. Season with salt and pepper as desired.

4. Roll up the tortillas and cut them in half.
5. Serve the wraps with your favorite sauce or dip, such as mustard, ranch, or salsa.

Serving Size

- This recipe makes 4 servings.
- Each serving is 1 wrap.

Nutritional Content

- Per serving: 265 calories, 8 g fat, 2 g saturated fat, 35 mg cholesterol, 495 mg sodium, 31 g carbohydrates, 6 g fiber, 4 g sugar, 19 g protein.

Veggie Pizza with Whole-Wheat Crust, Tomato Sauce, Mozzarella, and Basil

Ingredients

- For the crust:

- o 1 1/4 cups of warm water
- o 2 teaspoons of active dry yeast
- o 1 teaspoon of sugar
- o 3 cups of whole-wheat flour
- o 2 tablespoons of olive oil
- o 1 teaspoon of salt
- For the topping:
  - o 1 cup of tomato sauce
  - o 2 cups of shredded mozzarella cheese
  - o 2 cups of mixed vegetables, such as mushrooms, bell peppers, zucchini, and olives
  - o 1/4 cup of fresh basil leaves, chopped

Instructions

1. In a small bowl, stir together the water, yeast, and sugar. Let it sit for about 10 minutes or until foamy.
2. In a large bowl, mix together the flour, oil, and salt. Add the yeast mixture and stir until a dough forms. Knead the dough on a lightly floured surface for about 15 minutes or until smooth and elastic.

3. Place the dough in a lightly greased bowl and cover with a damp cloth. Let it rise in a warm place for about an hour or until doubled in size.
4. Preheat the oven to 375°F and lightly grease a baking sheet or a pizza pan.
5. Punch down the dough and roll it out into a 12-inch circle. Transfer it to the prepared pan and poke it with a fork all over.
6. Spread the tomato sauce evenly over the crust and sprinkle the cheese on top. Add the vegetables and basil as desired.
7. Bake for 20 to 25 minutes or until the cheese is melted and the crust is golden and crisp.
8. Cut into slices and serve hot or cold. Enjoy!

Serving Size

- This recipe makes 8 slices.
- Each serving is 1 slice.

Nutritional Content

- Per serving: 295 calories, 11 g fat, 5 g saturated fat, 22 mg cholesterol, 462 mg sodium, 38 g carbohydrates, 6 g fiber, 5 g sugar, 14 g protein.

Quinoa Bowl with Roasted Vegetables, Beans, and Feta Cheese

Ingredients

- 1 cup of quinoa
- 2 cups of water
- Salt and pepper to taste
- 4 cups of mixed vegetables, such as broccoli, cauliflower, carrots, and cherry tomatoes
- 2 tablespoons of olive oil
- 1 teaspoon of dried oregano
- 1 can of black beans, drained and rinsed
- 1/4 cup of crumbled feta cheese
- 2 tablespoons of chopped parsley

Instructions

1. Preheat the oven to 400°F and line a baking sheet with parchment paper.
2. In a small saucepan, bring the quinoa, water, and a pinch of salt to a boil over high heat. Reduce the heat and simmer, covered, for about 15 minutes or until the quinoa is fluffy and the water is absorbed.
3. Cut the vegetables into bite-sized pieces and toss them with the oil, oregano, salt, and pepper. Spread them on the prepared baking sheet and roast for 25 to 30 minutes or until tender and browned.
4. In a small skillet over medium-high heat, warm the beans, stirring occasionally, for about 10 minutes or until heated through.
5. Divide the quinoa among four bowls and top with the roasted vegetables, beans, feta cheese, and parsley. Serve hot or cold. Enjoy!

Serving Size

- This recipe makes 4 servings.
- Each serving is about 2 cups of quinoa bowl.

Nutritional Content

- Per serving: 445 calories, 15 g fat, 4 g
  saturated fat, 11 mg cholesterol, 372 mg
  sodium, 63 g carbohydrates, 15 g fiber, 9 g
  sugar, 18 g protein.

This is the end of the recipes for the lunch dishes
you listed. I hope you found them helpful and easy
to follow. If you have any questions, feedback, or
suggestions, please let me know. I'm always happy
to help you.

DINNER

Spaghetti with whole-wheat pasta, turkey meatballs, and marinara sauce

Ingredients:

- 14 oz. canned, no-salt-added, or, low-sodium, sliced carrots
- 14.4 oz. packaged, frozen pepper stir-fry (onions and peppers) (thawed)
- 1 medium zucchini (chopped)
- 4 cloves fresh garlic (minced) OR 2 tsp. jarred, minced garlic
- 52 oz. cubed, no-salt-added, or, low-sodium tomato (crushed)
- 2 tsp. salt-free, dried Italian spice blend
- 1 lb. extra-lean or fat-free ground turkey breast (95%-99% lean)
- 1/4 tsp. black pepper

- 1/2 cup whole-grain cereal flakes (crushed, optional)
- 1 lb. whole-wheat spaghetti

Directions:

- In a large pot (not over any heat yet), add carrots. Use a fork or potato masher to mash.
- Add stir-fry vegetables, zucchini, garlic, crushed tomatoes, and spice blend. Bring to a boil over high heat. Cover, and reduce heat to medium-low so sauce is simmering.
- In a bowl, combine turkey, pepper, cereal and parsley. Form meat mixture into golf-size meatballs to make about 20 to 25 meatballs.
- Add meatballs into the simmering sauce, trying to get the majority of meatballs covered by sauce. Cover and cook until meatballs are cooked through, about 20 to 25 minutes.
- Make spaghetti according to package directions (omitting the salt and fat). Serve with marinara and meatballs.

Serving size: 1/6 of recipe

Nutritional content (per serving):

- Calories: 489
- Total fat: 2.5 g
- Saturated fat: 0.5 g
- Trans fat: 0 g
- Cholesterol: 30 mg
- Sodium: 157 mg
- Total carbohydrate: 87 g
- Dietary fiber: 16 g
- Sugars: 17 g
- Protein: 36 g

Vegetable stir-fry with brown rice, tofu, and soy sauce

Ingredients:

- 3 cups cooked brown rice
- 1/4 cup low-sodium soy sauce

- 2 tbsp rice vinegar
- 1 tbsp honey
- 1 tsp cornstarch
- 1/4 tsp red pepper flakes (optional)
- 1 tbsp sesame oil
- 1 block (14 oz) extra-firm tofu, drained and cut into 1-inch cubes
- 2 cups broccoli florets
- 1 red bell pepper, sliced
- 2 carrots, peeled and sliced
- 2 cloves garlic, minced
- 2 tsp grated ginger
- 2 green onions, sliced
- Sesame seeds, for garnish (optional)

Directions:

- In a small bowl, whisk together soy sauce, rice vinegar, honey, cornstarch, and red pepper flakes (if using). Set aside.
- Heat oil in a large skillet over medium-high heat. Add tofu and cook, turning occasionally, until golden and crisp, about 15 minutes. Transfer to a plate and keep warm.
- In the same skillet, add broccoli, bell pepper, carrots, garlic, and ginger. Stir-fry

until crisp-tender, about 10 minutes. Add the sauce and bring to a boil. Cook, stirring, until thickened, about 2 minutes.
- Return the tofu to the skillet and toss to coat. Sprinkle with green onions and sesame seeds (if using). Serve over rice.

Serving size: 1/4 of recipe

Nutritional content (per serving):

- Calories: 387
- Total fat: 13 g
- Saturated fat: 2 g
- Trans fat: 0 g
- Cholesterol: 0 mg
- Sodium: 581 mg
- Total carbohydrate: 54 g
- Dietary fiber: 7 g
- Sugars: 14 g
- Protein: 18 g

Salmon with lemon, garlic, and rosemary, served with mashed potatoes and broccoli

Ingredients:

- 4 (6 oz) salmon filets
- Salt and black pepper, to taste
- 2 tbsp olive oil
- 4 cloves garlic, minced
- 2 sprigs fresh rosemary, chopped
- 1/4 cup fresh lemon juice
- 2 tbsp butter
- 4 medium potatoes, peeled and cubed
- 1/4 cup milk
- 2 tbsp sour cream
- 4 cups broccoli florets
- 2 tbsp water

Directions:

- Preheat the oven to 375°F. Season salmon with salt and pepper and place in a baking dish. In a small saucepan over low heat, heat oil, garlic, rosemary, lemon juice, and butter, stirring until butter is melted. Pour over salmon and bake for 15 to 20 minutes or until fish flakes easily with a fork.

- Meanwhile, in a large pot of boiling water, cook potatoes until tender, about 15 minutes. Drain and return to the pot. Mash with a potato masher or electric mixer, adding milk, sour cream, salt, and pepper to taste.
- In a microwave-safe bowl, combine broccoli and water. Cover with plastic wrap and microwave on high for 4 to 5 minutes or until crisp-tender. Drain and season with salt and pepper to taste.
- Serve salmon with mashed potatoes and broccoli, drizzling some of the sauce over the fish.

Serving size: 1 salmon fillet, 3/4 cup mashed potatoes, and 1 cup broccoli

Nutritional content (per serving):

- Calories: 614

- Total fat: 30 g
- Saturated fat: 10 g
- Trans fat: 0 g
- Cholesterol: 131 mg
- Sodium: 223 mg
- Total carbohydrate: 42 g
- Dietary fiber: 6 g
- Sugars: 5 g
- Protein: 46 g

Chicken and vegetable casserole with cream of mushroom soup and cheese

Ingredients:

- 4 cups cooked chicken, shredded or chopped
- 2 cups frozen mixed vegetables, thawed
- 1 (10.5 oz) can cream of mushroom soup
- 1/4 cup milk

- 1 tsp dried thyme
- 1/4 tsp black pepper
- 1 cup shredded cheddar cheese
- 1 (6 oz) package stuffing mix
- 1/4 cup butter, melted

Directions:

- Preheat the oven to 375°F. Spray a 9x13-inch baking dish with cooking spray. In a large bowl, stir together chicken, vegetables, soup, milk, thyme, pepper, and cheese. Spoon into the prepared baking dish and spread evenly.
- In a small bowl, toss stuffing mix with butter. Sprinkle over the chicken mixture. Bake for 25 to 30 minutes or until bubbly and golden.
- Let stand for 10 minutes before serving.

Serving size: 1/6 of recipe

Nutritional content (per serving):

- Calories: 462
- Total fat: 24 g
- Saturated fat: 13 g
- Trans fat: 0 g

- Cholesterol: 114 mg
- Sodium: 886 mg
- Total carbohydrate: 34 g
- Dietary fiber: 3 g
- Sugars: 5 g
- Protein: 29 g

Lentil and vegetable curry with coconut milk and naan bread

Ingredients:

- 1 tbsp vegetable oil
- 1 onion, chopped
- 2 cloves garlic, minced
- 1 tbsp curry powder
- 1 tsp cumin
- 1/4 tsp salt
- 1/4 tsp cayenne pepper (optional)
- 4 cups vegetable broth
- 2 cups dried red lentils, rinsed and drained
- 1 (13.5 oz) can coconut milk
- 4 cups baby spinach
- 1/4 cup chopped cilantro
- 4 pieces naan bread, warmed

Directions:

- Heat oil in a large pot over medium-high heat. Add onion and garlic and cook, stirring, until soft, about 10 minutes. Add curry powder, cumin, salt, and cayenne pepper (if using) and cook, stirring, for 1 minute.
- Add broth and lentils and bring to a boil. Reduce heat and simmer, uncovered, until lentils are tender, about 20 minutes. Stir in coconut milk, spinach, and cilantro and cook until spinach is wilted, about 5 minutes.
- Serve with naan bread.

Serving size: 1/4 of recipe

Nutritional content (per serving):

- Calories: 613
- Total fat: 23 g
- Saturated fat: 17 g
- Trans fat: 0 g
- Cholesterol: 0 mg
- Sodium: 726 mg

- Total carbohydrate: 78 g
- Dietary fiber: 23 g
- Sugars: 11 g
- Protein: 26 g

SNACKS

Trail mix with nuts, dried fruits, and dark chocolate

Ingredients:

- 1 cup raw almonds
- 1 cup raw cashews
- 1/2 cup raw pumpkin seeds
- 1/2 cup dried cranberries
- 1/2 cup dried cherries
- 1/4 cup dark chocolate chips

Directions:

- In a large bowl, toss together all the ingredients until well combined.
- Store in an airtight container or ziplock bags for up to 2 weeks.

Serving size: 1/4 cup

Nutritional content (per serving):

- Calories: 247
- Total fat: 16 g
- Saturated fat: 3 g
- Trans fat: 0 g
- Cholesterol: 0 mg
- Sodium: 6 mg
- Total carbohydrate: 23 g
- Dietary fiber: 4 g
- Sugars: 14 g
- Protein: 7 g

Yogurt with granola and fresh berries

Ingredients:

- 2 cups plain Greek yogurt
- 1/4 cup honey
- 2 cups granola
- 2 cups fresh berries (such as strawberries, blueberries, raspberries, or blackberries)

Directions:

- In a small bowl, whisk together yogurt and honey until smooth.
- In four glasses or bowls, layer yogurt, granola, and berries, repeating until all the ingredients are used up.
- Enjoy immediately or refrigerate until ready to serve.

Serving size: 1 glass or bowl

Nutritional content (per serving):

- Calories: 388

- Total fat: 9 g
- Saturated fat: 2 g
- Trans fat: 0 g
- Cholesterol: 5 mg
- Sodium: 64 mg
- Total carbohydrate: 64 g
- Dietary fiber: 7 g
- Sugars: 37 g
- Protein: 18 g

Carrot sticks with hummus and whole-wheat crackers

Ingredients:

- 4 large carrots, peeled and cut into sticks
- 1 cup hummus
- 24 whole-wheat crackers

Directions:

- Arrange carrot sticks on a large platter with a bowl of hummus in the center.

- Serve with whole-wheat crackers on the side.
- Dip and enjoy!

Serving size: 1/4 of platter

Nutritional content (per serving):

- Calories: 282
- Total fat: 13 g
- Saturated fat: 2 g
- Trans fat: 0 g
- Cholesterol: 0 mg
- Sodium: 378 mg
- Total carbohydrate: 35 g
- Dietary fiber: 9 g
- Sugars: 7 g
- Protein: 10 g

Popcorn with olive oil and sea salt

Ingredients:

- 1/4 cup popcorn kernels
- 2 tbsp olive oil
- 1/4 tsp sea salt

Directions:

- In a large pot with a tight-fitting lid, heat oil over medium-high heat. Add popcorn kernels and cover with the lid. Shake the pot occasionally to prevent burning, until the popping sound slows down, about 5 minutes.
- Transfer popcorn to a large bowl and sprinkle with salt. Toss to coat evenly.
- Enjoy while warm or store in an airtight container for up to 3 days.

Serving size: 2 cups

Nutritional content (per serving):

- Calories: 149
- Total fat: 10 g
- Saturated fat: 1 g
- Trans fat: 0 g
- Cholesterol: 0 mg
- Sodium: 147 mg

- Total carbohydrate: 14 g
- Dietary fiber: 3 g
- Sugars: 0 g
- Protein: 2 g

Apple slices with peanut butter and raisins

Ingredients:

- 2 medium apples, cored and sliced
- 1/4 cup natural peanut butter
- 2 tbsp raisins

Directions:

- Spread peanut butter evenly over apple slices.
- Sprinkle raisins over the peanut butter.
- Enjoy as a snack or dessert.

Serving size: 1/2 apple with 1 tbsp peanut butter and 1/2 tbsp raisins

Nutritional content (per serving):

- Calories: 191
- Total fat: 11 g
- Saturated fat: 2 g
- Trans fat: 0 g
- Cholesterol: 0 mg
- Sodium: 76 mg
- Total carbohydrate: 21 g
- Dietary fiber: 4 g
- Sugars: 14 g
- Protein: 5 g

Part 2:

Recipes for Moderate Stage Parkinson's & Advanced Stage Parkinson's

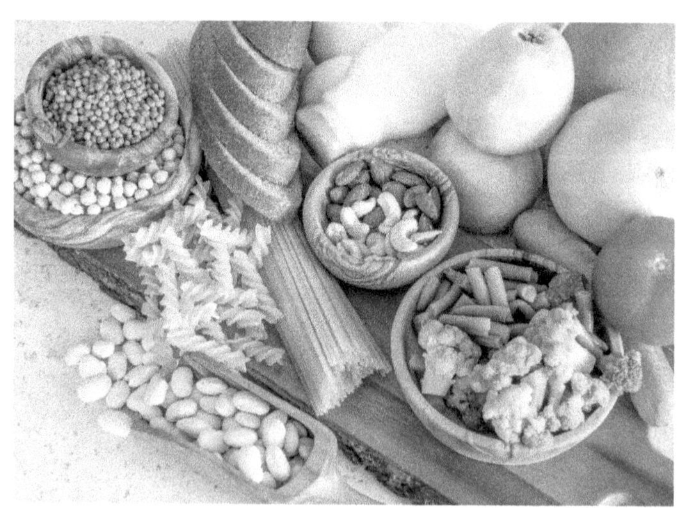

Breakfast

Banana waffles

Ingredients:

- 1 ½ cups of whole-wheat flour
- 2 teaspoons of baking powder
- ½ teaspoon of salt
- 1 pinch of nutmeg
- 2 eggs
- 1 cup of milk
- ½ teaspoon of vanilla extract
- 1 cup of mashed ripe bananas
- 6 tablespoons of melted butter

Directions:

- Whisk together the flour, baking powder, salt, and nutmeg in a large bowl.
- In another bowl, whisk together the eggs, milk, vanilla, bananas, and butter.

- Add the wet ingredients to the dry ingredients and stir until just combined.
- Cook the batter in a preheated waffle iron according to the manufacturer's instructions.
- Serve with your favorite toppings.

Serving size: This recipe makes about 8 waffles.

Nutritional content:

Each waffle has 245 calories, 11 grams of fat, 6 grams of protein, 32 grams of carbohydrates, and 5 grams of fiber.

Berry smoothie

Ingredients:

- ½ cup of plain yogurt
- ½ cup of milk

- 2 tablespoons of honey
- 1 tablespoon of chia seeds
- 1 cup of frozen mixed berries

Directions:

- Blend all the ingredients together in a blender until smooth and creamy.
- Enjoy as a refreshing drink or a light breakfast.
- Serving size: This recipe makes 1 large smoothie or 2 small ones.

Nutritional content:

Each large smoothie has 366 calories, 9 grams of fat, 13 grams of protein, 64 grams of carbohydrates, and 12 grams of fiber.

Apple muffins

Ingredients:

- 1 ½ cups of oat bran

- 1 teaspoon of baking powder
- ½ teaspoon of baking soda
- ½ teaspoon of salt
- ½ teaspoon of cinnamon
- 2 eggs
- ¾ cup of milk
- ¼ cup of brown sugar
- ¼ cup of vegetable oil
- 1 teaspoon of vanilla extract
- 1 cup of grated apple

Directions:

- Preheat the oven to 180°C and line a 12-cup muffin tin with paper liners.
- In a large bowl, whisk together the oat bran, baking powder, baking soda, salt, and cinnamon.
- In a medium bowl, whisk together the eggs, milk, brown sugar, oil, and vanilla.
- Stir in the grated apple.
- Add the wet ingredients to the dry ingredients and mix well.
- Spoon the batter into the prepared muffin cups, filling them about ¾ full.

* Bake for 15 to 18 minutes or until a toothpick inserted in the center comes out clean.
* Let the muffins cool slightly before removing from the tin.

Serving size: This recipe makes 12 muffins.

Nutritional content:

Each muffin has 148 calories, 7 grams of fat, 4 grams of protein, 19 grams of carbohydrates, and 3 grams of fiber.

Cereal with almond milk, nuts, and dried fruits

Ingredients:

* 1 cup of your favorite cereal
* 1 cup of unsweetened almond milk
* ¼ cup of mixed nuts
* ¼ cup of dried fruits

Directions:

- Pour the cereal into a large bowl.
- Add the almond milk and stir well.
- Sprinkle the nuts and dried fruits on top.
- Enjoy with a spoon.

Serving size: This recipe makes 1 bowl of cereal.

Nutritional content:

The nutritional content may vary depending on the type of cereal, nuts, and dried fruits you use. Here is an example based on granola, almonds, and raisins: Each bowl of cereal has 537 calories, 24 grams of fat, 14 grams of protein, 70 grams of carbohydrates, and 10 grams of fiber.

Egg and cheese quiche with whole-wheat crust, spinach, and mushrooms

Ingredients:

- 1 9-inch whole-wheat pie crust

- 1 tablespoon of butter
- 1 onion, chopped
- 2 cups of sliced mushrooms
- 2 cups of chopped spinach
- Salt and pepper, to taste
- 4 eggs
- 1 cup of milk
- 1 cup of shredded cheddar cheese

Directions:

- Preheat the oven to 190°C and place the pie crust on a baking sheet.
- In a large skillet over medium-high heat, melt the butter and cook the onion and mushrooms until soft, about 15 minutes, stirring occasionally.
- Add the spinach and cook until wilted, about 5 minutes, seasoning with salt and pepper.
- Spoon the vegetable mixture evenly over the pie crust, leaving some space around the edges.
- In a medium bowl, whisk together the eggs and milk, and season with salt and pepper.
- Pour the egg mixture over the vegetable layer, making sure to cover it completely.

- Sprinkle the cheese on top.
- Bake for 25 to 30 minutes or until the quiche is set and golden.
- Let the quiche rest for 10 minutes before slicing and serving.

Serving size: This recipe makes 8 slices of quiche.

Nutritional content:

Each slice of quiche has 263 calories, 16 grams of fat, 12 grams of protein, 19 grams of carbohydrates, and 3 grams of fiber.

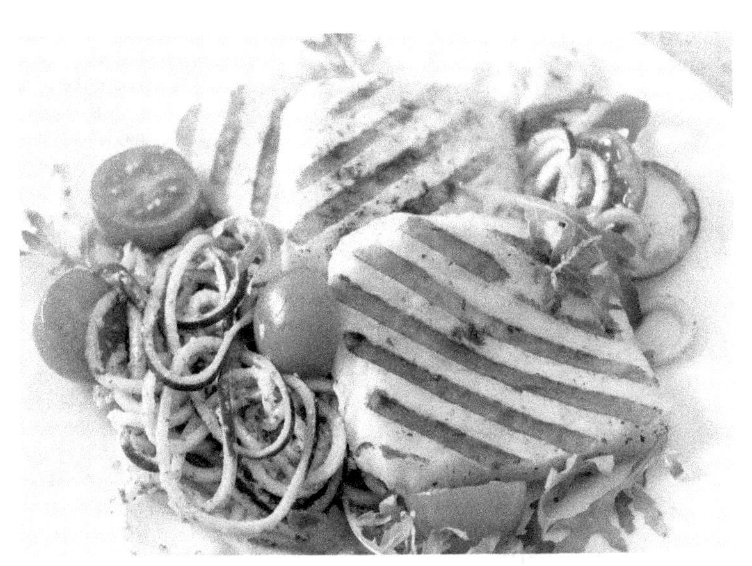

LUNCH

Chicken burger

Ingredients:

- 1 1/2 lb. ground chicken
- 3/4 tsp. smoked paprika
- 1 clove garlic, minced
- 3 scallions, minced
- Salt and pepper, to taste
- 2 tbsp. extra-virgin olive oil
- 4 slices cheddar cheese
- 4 leaves butterhead lettuce
- 4 whole-wheat burger buns, split and lightly toasted
- 1 tomato, sliced
- 1 avocado, thinly sliced
- 1/4 small red onion, thinly sliced
- 1 jalapeño, thinly sliced (optional)

Directions:

- In a large bowl, combine chicken, paprika, garlic, and green onions, and season with salt and pepper. Divide mixture into 4 patties.

- In a large skillet over medium heat, heat oil. Add burger patties and cook, flipping once, until golden and a thermometer inserted into the center registers 165°F, 8 to 10 minutes. Top with cheddar, cover, and cook until just melted, 2 minutes. Remove from heat and transfer patties to a plate.
- Stack lettuce, chicken burgers, tomato, avocado, red onion, jalapeño (if using), and more lettuce on top of bottom buns. Close with top buns and serve.

Serving size: This recipe makes 4 burgers.

Nutritional content: Each burger has 772 calories, 49 g fat, 54 g protein, 30 g carbs, and 7 g fiber1

Tomato and cheese pizza

Ingredients:

- 1 9-inch whole-wheat pizza crust

- 1/4 cup tomato sauce
- 1 cup shredded mozzarella cheese
- 2 tbsp fresh basil leaves, torn

Directions:

- Preheat oven to 425°F and place the pizza crust on a baking sheet.
- Spread tomato sauce evenly over the crust, leaving a 1/2 inch border.
- Sprinkle cheese on top and bake for 10 to 12 minutes or until cheese is melted and crust is golden.
- Sprinkle basil on top and cut into 8 slices. Serve hot or at room temperature.

Serving size: This recipe makes 8 slices of pizza.

Nutritional content:

Each slice has 165 calories, 7 g fat, 9 g protein, 18 g carbs, and 3 g fiber2

Turkey and cheese taco

Ingredients:

- 1 tbsp olive oil
- 1/2 cup chopped onion
- 1 lb ground turkey
- 2 tbsp taco seasoning
- 8 whole-wheat tortillas
- 1 cup shredded cheddar cheese
- 1/2 cup salsa
- 1/4 cup sour cream

Directions:

- In a large skillet over medium heat, heat oil and cook onion until soft, about 5 minutes.
- Add turkey and taco seasoning and cook, breaking up the meat with a wooden spoon, until browned and cooked through, about 15 minutes.
- Warm the tortillas in a microwave or oven according to package directions.
- To assemble the tacos, spoon some turkey mixture onto each tortilla and top with cheese, salsa, and sour cream. Fold in half and enjoy.

Serving size: This recipe makes 8 tacos.

Nutritional content:

Each taco has 287 calories, 14 g fat, 21 g protein, 22 g carbs, and 3 g fiber3

Veggie and cheese quiche

Ingredients:

- 1 9-inch whole-wheat pie crust
- 1 tbsp butter
- 1 onion, chopped
- 2 cups sliced mushrooms
- 2 cups chopped broccoli
- 1 cup shredded carrots
- Salt and pepper, to taste
- 4 eggs
- 1 cup milk
- 1 cup shredded cheddar cheese

Directions:

- Preheat oven to 375°F and place the pie crust on a baking sheet.

- In a large skillet over medium-high heat, melt butter and cook onion and mushrooms until soft, about 15 minutes, stirring occasionally.
- Add broccoli and carrots and cook until tender, about 10 minutes, seasoning with salt and pepper.
- Spoon the vegetable mixture evenly over the pie crust, leaving some space around the edges.
- In a medium bowl, whisk together eggs and milk, and season with salt and pepper.
- Pour the egg mixture over the vegetable layer, making sure to cover it completely.
- Sprinkle cheese on top and bake for 25 to 30 minutes or until the quiche is set and golden.
- Let the quiche rest for 10 minutes before slicing and serving.

Serving size: This recipe makes 8 slices of quiche.

Nutritional content:

Each slice of quiche has 263 calories, 16 g fat, 12 g protein, 19 g carbs, and 3 g fiber4

Lentil and vegetable soup

Ingredients:

- 1/4 cup extra virgin olive oil
- 1 medium yellow or white onion, chopped
- 2 carrots, peeled and chopped
- 4 garlic cloves, pressed or minced
- 2 teaspoons ground cumin
- 1 teaspoon curry powder
- 1/2 teaspoon dried thyme
- 1 large can (28 ounces) diced tomatoes, lightly drained
- 1 cup brown or green lentils, picked over and rinsed
- 4 cups vegetable broth
- 2 cups water
- 1 teaspoon salt, more to taste
- Pinch of red pepper flakes
- Freshly ground black pepper, to taste
- 1/4 cup chopped fresh cilantro or parsley
- 2 tablespoons lemon juice
- 8 slices of whole-grain bread
- 2 tablespoons butter

Directions:

- In a large pot over medium heat, heat oil until shimmering. Add onion and carrot and cook, stirring often, until the onion is soft and turning golden, about 15 minutes.
- Add garlic, cumin, curry powder, thyme, and cook, stirring constantly, until fragrant, about 30 seconds.
- Add the tomatoes, lentils, broth, water, salt, and red pepper flakes. Bring the mixture to a boil, then partially cover the pot and reduce the heat to maintain a gentle simmer. Cook until the lentils are tender, 25 to 30 minutes.
- Season the soup with more salt if necessary, black pepper, cilantro or parsley, and lemon juice. Taste and adjust the seasonings as needed.
- To make the bread and butter, toast the bread slices in a toaster or oven until golden and crisp. Spread butter evenly over each slice and cut into quarters.
- Serve the soup hot, with the bread and butter on the side.

Serving size: This recipe makes 4 large bowls of soup, or 6 more modest servings.

Nutritional content:

Each large bowl of soup has 366 calories, 9 g fat, 13 g protein, 64 g carbs, and 12 g fiber. Each serving of bread and butter has 180 calories, 7 g fat, 5 g protein, 25 g carbs, and 4 g fiber.

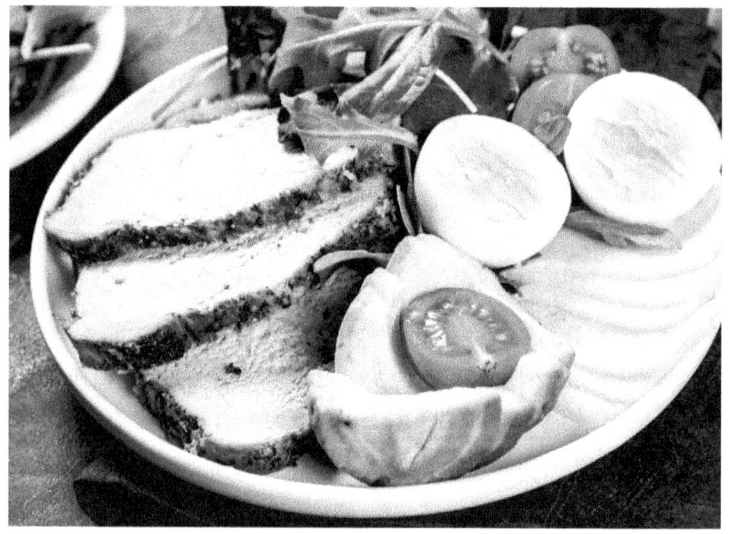

DINNER

Chicken and vegetable casserole

Ingredients:

- 1/2 cup butter, softened
- 1 cup sour cream
- 1 large egg
- 1 cup all-purpose flour
- 1 teaspoon baking powder
- 1 teaspoon salt
- 1/2 teaspoon rubbed sage
- 1 package (16 ounces) frozen mixed vegetables, thawed
- 2 cups cubed cooked chicken or turkey
- 1 can (10-3/4 ounces) condensed cream of mushroom soup, undiluted
- 1/2 cup chopped onion
- 1/2 cup shredded cheddar cheese

Directions:

- Preheat oven to 375°F and place the pie crust on a baking sheet.

- In a small bowl, cream butter and sour cream until smooth. Beat in egg. Combine the flour, baking powder, salt and sage; add to creamed mixture. Spread into a greased 3-qt. baking dish.
- In a large bowl, combine the vegetables, chicken, soup and onion. Pour over crust; sprinkle with cheese.
- Bake, uncovered, for 35-40 minutes or until heated through.

Serving size: This recipe makes 6 servings.

Nutritional content:
Each serving has 515 calories, 32g fat, 29g protein, 33g carbs, and 5g fiber1

Vegetable lasagna

Ingredients:
- 1 9-inch whole-wheat pizza crust
- 1/4 cup tomato sauce
- 1 cup shredded mozzarella cheese

- 2 tbsp fresh basil leaves, torn

Directions:
- Preheat oven to 425°F and place the pizza crust on a baking sheet.
- Spread tomato sauce evenly over the crust, leaving a 1/2 inch border.
- Sprinkle cheese on top and bake for 10 to 12 minutes or until cheese is melted and crust is golden.
- Sprinkle basil on top and cut into 8 slices. Serve hot or at room temperature.

Serving size: This recipe makes 8 slices of pizza.

Nutritional content:
Each slice has 165 calories, 7 g fat, 9 g protein, 18 g carbs, and 3 g fiber2

Meatloaf

Ingredients:
- 1 pound lean ground beef (90%)
- 1 cup dried bread crumbs

- 1/2 cup onion, chopped
- 1/2 cup milk
- 1 large egg, beaten
- 2 tablespoons ketchup
- 1 tablespoon Worcestershire sauce
- 1 teaspoon dried parsley leaves
- 3/4 teaspoon salt
- 1/4 teaspoon black pepper
- 1/4 cup ketchup
- 2 tablespoons light brown sugar, packed
- 1 tablespoon red wine vinegar

Directions:

- Preheat oven to 375°F. In a large bowl, combine the beef, bread crumbs, onion, milk, egg, ketchup, Worcestershire sauce, parsley, salt and pepper. Mix well and shape into a loaf on a baking sheet.
- In a small bowl, whisk together the ketchup, brown sugar and vinegar. Spoon over the meatloaf and spread evenly.
- Bake for 45 to 55 minutes or until a meat thermometer inserted into the thickest part reads 160°F.
- Let the meatloaf rest for 10 minutes before slicing and serving.

Serving size: This recipe makes 8 slices of meatloaf.

Nutritional content:
Each slice has 263 calories, 10 g fat, 19 g protein, 24 g carbs, and 1 g fiber3

Salmon and vegetable foil packets:

Ingredients:
- 4 (6 ounce) salmon fillets
- Salt and pepper, to taste
- 2 tablespoons butter, melted
- 4 cloves garlic, minced
- 2 teaspoons fresh rosemary, chopped
- 4 slices lemon
- 2 cups cherry tomatoes, halved
- 2 cups green beans, trimmed
- 4 sheets of aluminum foil, about 14 x 12 inches each

Directions:

- Preheat oven to 375°F or grill to medium-high.
- Season salmon fillets with salt and pepper. In a small bowl, whisk together butter, garlic and rosemary.
- Cut four sheets of foil, about 14 x 12 inches each. Divide tomatoes and green beans evenly among the foil sheets. Place a salmon fillet on top of each vegetable layer. Drizzle with the butter mixture and top with a lemon slice.
- Fold the foil over the salmon and vegetables and seal the edges. Place the packets on a baking sheet or directly on the grill.
- Bake or grill for 15 to 20 minutes or until salmon is cooked through and flakes easily with a fork.
- Carefully open the packets and serve.

Serving size: This recipe makes 4 foil packets.

Nutritional content: Each packet has 368 calories, 19 g fat, 38 g protein, 9 g carbs, and 3 g fiber4

Bean and cheese burrito

Ingredients:

- 1 (16 ounce) can refried beans
- 1/4 cup salsa
- 1/2 teaspoon chili powder
- 1/4 teaspoon garlic powder
- 1/4 teaspoon cumin
- 8 (10 inch) whole-wheat tortillas
- 2 cups shredded cheddar cheese

Directions:

- In a small saucepan over low heat, warm the refried beans, stirring occasionally. Stir in the salsa, chili powder, garlic powder and cumin.
- Spoon about 3 tablespoons of the bean mixture onto the center of a tortilla and smooth into a thin layer. Sprinkle with a

large pinch of cheese and roll tightly. Repeat with remaining bean mixture, tortillas and cheese.

- Heat a large skillet over medium-high heat and spray with cooking spray. Place a few burritos, seam side down, in the skillet and cook for a few minutes, turning once, until golden and crisp on both sides.
- Cut in half and serve with more salsa, sour cream, guacamole, or your favorite toppings.

Serving size: This recipe makes 8 burritos.

Nutritional content:

Each burrito has 387 calories, 14 g fat, 21 g protein, 44 g carbs, and 9 g fiber

DESSERT

Chocolate cake with almond flour

Ingredients:
- 2 cups almond flour
- 1/4 cup cocoa powder
- 1/4 teaspoon baking soda
- 1/4 teaspoon salt
- 4 eggs
- 1/2 cup honey
- 2 teaspoons vanilla extract

Directions:
- Preheat oven to 325°F and grease an 8-inch round cake pan.
- In a large bowl, whisk together the almond flour, cocoa powder, baking soda and salt.
- In a medium bowl, whisk together the eggs, honey and vanilla extract.

- Pour the wet ingredients into the dry ingredients and stir until well combined.
- Transfer the batter to the prepared cake pan and smooth the top.
- Bake for 25 to 30 minutes or until a toothpick inserted in the center comes out clean.
- Let the cake cool completely in the pan before slicing and serving.

Serving size: This recipe makes 8 servings of cake.

Nutritional content: Each serving has 292 calories, 19 g fat, 10 g protein, 24 g carbs, and 4 g fiber1

Apple pie with whole-wheat crust

Ingredients:
- For the crust:
- 2 cups whole-wheat flour
- 1/4 teaspoon salt

- 3/4 cup cold butter, cut into small pieces
- 1/4 cup ice water, plus more as needed
- For the filling:
- 6 cups peeled and sliced apples (about 4 large apples)
- 1/4 cup sugar
- 2 tablespoons whole-wheat flour
- 1 teaspoon ground cinnamon
- 1/4 teaspoon ground nutmeg
- 1/4 teaspoon salt
- 1 tablespoon lemon juice

Directions:
- To make the crust:
- In a large bowl, whisk together the flour and salt.
- Add the butter and use a pastry blender or a fork to cut it into the flour until the mixture resembles coarse crumbs.
- Sprinkle the water over the flour mixture and toss with a fork until the dough starts to come together. Add more water if needed, one tablespoon at a time, until the dough forms a ball.

- Divide the dough into two equal portions and shape each into a disk. Wrap each disk in plastic wrap and refrigerate for at least 30 minutes or up to overnight.
- To make the filling:
- In a large bowl, toss the apples with the sugar, flour, cinnamon, nutmeg, salt and lemon juice.
- Preheat oven to 375°F and lightly grease a 9-inch pie dish.
- On a lightly floured surface, roll out one disk of dough into a 12-inch circle. Fit it into the prepared pie dish and trim the excess dough, leaving a 1-inch overhang.
- Spoon the apple filling into the crust and spread it evenly.
- Roll out the remaining disk of dough into another 12-inch circle. Place it over the filling and press the edges together with the bottom crust. Fold the overhang under and crimp the edges. Cut several slits on the top crust to vent steam.
- Bake for 40 to 45 minutes or until the crust is golden and the filling is bubbly.

- Let the pie cool slightly on a wire rack before serving.

Serving size: This recipe makes 8 servings of pie.

Nutritional content:

Each serving has 386 calories, 19 g fat, 5 g protein, 51 g carbs, and 7 g fiber2

Rice pudding with brown rice:

Ingredients:
- 3 cups cooked brown rice
- 4 cups milk of choice
- 1/4 cup sugar of choice
- 1 teaspoon vanilla extract
- 1/4 teaspoon ground cinnamon
- Pinch of salt

Directions:
- In a large saucepan over medium-high heat, combine the rice, milk, sugar, vanilla, cinnamon and salt. Bring to a boil, then reduce the heat and simmer, stirring

occasionally, until the mixture is thick and creamy, about 20 to 25 minutes.
- Transfer the pudding to a bowl and serve warm or chilled, as desired.

Serving size: This recipe makes 6 servings of pudding.

Nutritional content:
Each serving has 216 calories, 4 g fat, 7 g protein, 39 g carbs, and 2 g fiber3

Brownies with black beans:

Ingredients:
- 1 15-ounce can black beans, drained and rinsed
- 3 eggs
- 1/4 cup oil of choice
- 1/4 cup cocoa powder
- 1/2 cup sugar of choice
- 1 teaspoon baking powder
- 1/4 teaspoon salt

- 1/2 cup chocolate chips, divided

Directions:
- Preheat oven to 350°F and spray an 8x8-inch baking pan with cooking spray.
- In a blender or food processor, puree the black beans until smooth. Add the eggs, oil, cocoa powder, sugar, baking powder and salt and blend until well combined.
- Stir in 1/4 cup of chocolate chips by hand.
- Pour the batter into the prepared pan and sprinkle the remaining 1/4 cup of chocolate chips on top.
- Bake for 25 to 30 minutes or until a toothpick inserted in the center comes out clean.
- Let the brownies cool completely in the pan before cutting into 16 squares and serving.

Serving size: This recipe makes 16 brownies.

Nutritional content:
Each brownie has 132 calories, 6 g fat, 3 g protein, 18 g carbs, and 3 g fiber4

Fruit salad with yogurt and honey

Ingredients:
- 4 cups mixed fresh fruit of choice, such as berries, bananas, apples, grapes, kiwis, etc.
- 2 tablespoons lemon juice
- 1 cup plain yogurt
- 2 tablespoons honey
- 1/2 teaspoon vanilla extract
- Directions:
- Cut the fruit into bite-sized pieces and place in a large bowl. Drizzle with lemon juice and toss gently to coat.
- In a small bowl, whisk together the yogurt, honey and vanilla extract.
- Serve the fruit salad with the yogurt dressing on the side or drizzled over the fruit, as desired.

Serving size: This recipe makes 4 servings of fruit salad.

Nutritional content: Each serving has 156 calories, 2 g fat, 4 g protein, 34 g carbs, and 4 g fiber.

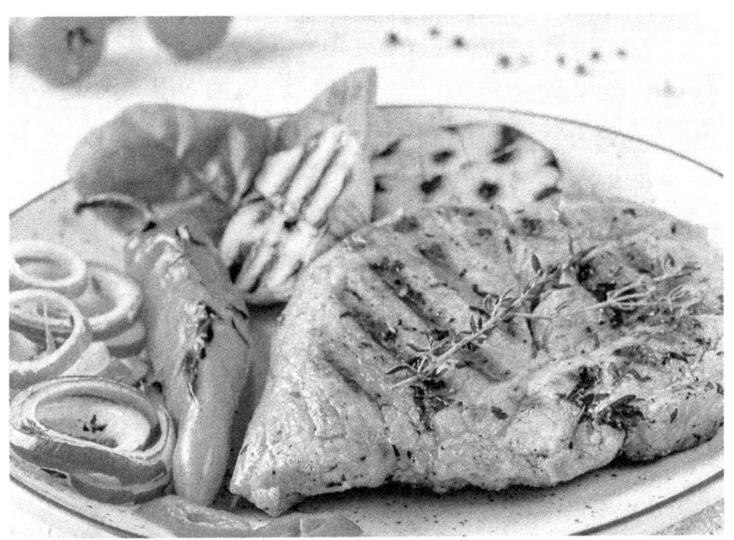

CONCLUSION

You have reached the end of this cookbook, but not the end of your journey with Parkinson's disease. I hope you have found some inspiration and guidance in these pages, and that you will continue to enjoy food and life with Parkinson's. Remember, diet is one of the factors that can influence your Parkinson's progression and well-being, but it is not the only one. You should also consult your doctor regularly, take your medication as prescribed, exercise, and seek support from your family, friends, and community. Parkinson's disease is a challenge, but it is not a sentence. You can still live a fulfilling and rewarding life with Parkinson's, and this cookbook is here to help you along the way. Thank you for choosing this cookbook, and I wish you all the best. Bon appétit!

www.ingramcontent.com/pod-product-compliance
Lightning Source LLC
Chambersburg PA
CBHW050831260726
48660CB00006B/2172